Pub 1985

# DOCTOR at DUNKIRK

*What though the field be lost?*
*All is not lost.*

MILTON
Paradise Lost

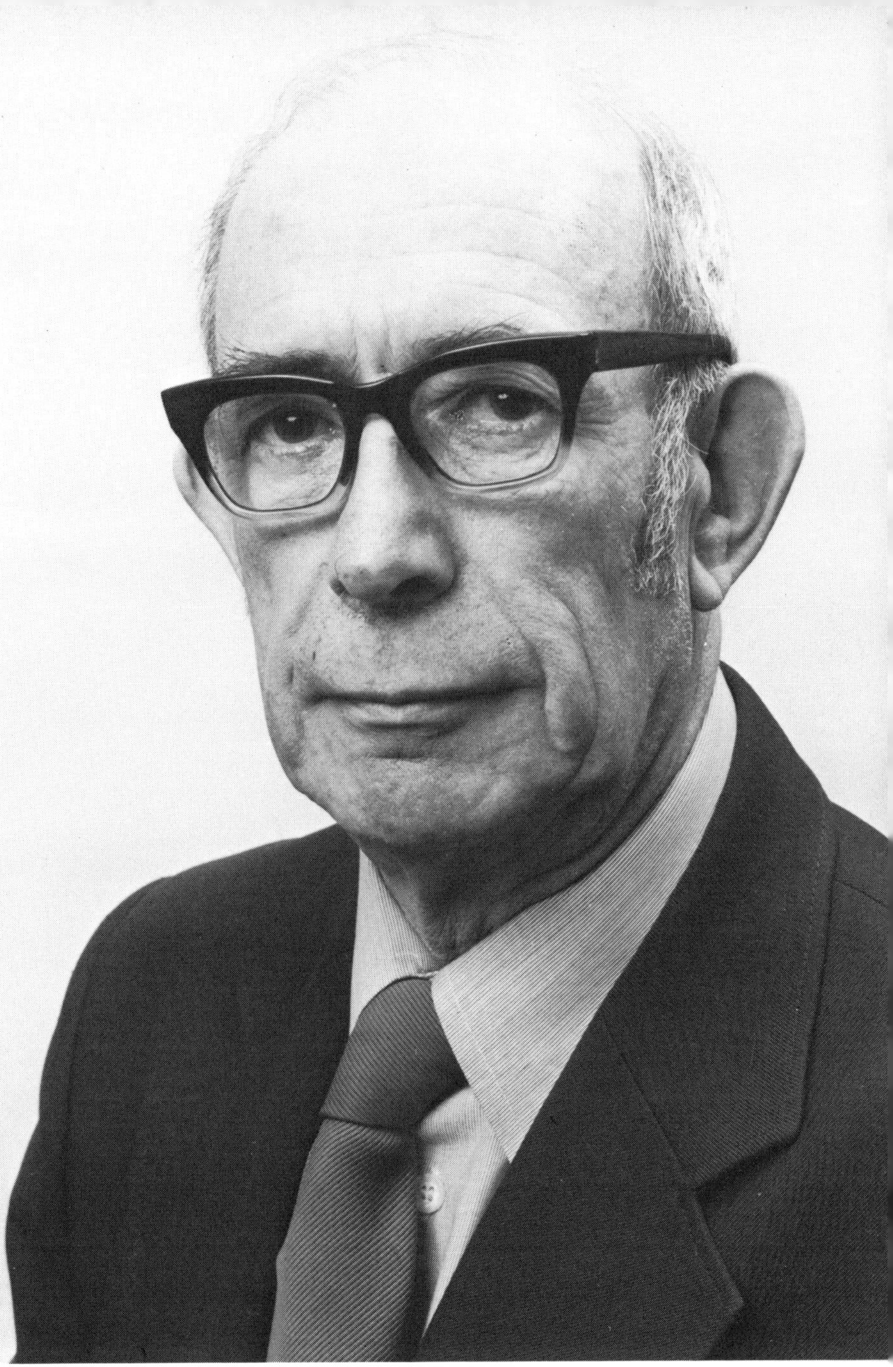

*Ian Samuel*

# DOCTOR at DUNKIRK

## with the 6th Field Ambulance at war

IAN SAMUEL
OBE, MRCS, LRCP, D Obst, RCOG

Autolycus Publications
1985

Phototypesetting by Aquarian Typesetters,
London WC2

ISBN: 0 903413 75 2

Published by Autolycus Publications
14 Barlby Road London W10 6AR
in association with Triad Press.

# Contents

*This short episode of war experience is dedicated to Joy, who had the incomparably more difficult job of bringing up our children under wartime conditions.*

# Introduction and Acknowledgements

In no way is this the full story of 6th Field Ambulance, but the memories of the shattering impact of some eighteen days in the life of a general medical practitioner in particular from May 10th, 1940 onwards. I am indebted to many ranks from the unit who have refreshed my memory as to events some forty-five years ago, and to personal accounts that some of them had written for a small booklet for the unit's Old Comrade Association of their journeys from France to Burma via Dunkirk. My special thanks to Sergeant Eric Knight, George Nightingale and Reg Hales for invaluable help. As all my fellow Officers with the unit during the relevant period have, alas, died, I — in my seventy-ninth year — have had to speak for them. I hope they will forgive me.

My thanks are due to the Imperial War Museum and the Public Record Office for much help and courtesy. But above all I should like to thank my editor, Lewis Foreman, for dragging this story from me and then helping me put it into some sort of order.

IAN SAMUEL

# I

In the Summer of 1939 it seemed obvious to everybody that we should be at war with Germany in the very near future, so I decided to apply for a Commission in the Supplementary Reserve of the Royal Army Medical Corps. After interviews I was told I would be Commissioned on September 19th, 1939. I asked what my position was should war break out before that date and was informed that the date would still be the 19th September before I would be in the RAMC, and that is what happened.

The day after war broke out I was telephoned by a patient of mine who was a territorial soldier on duty at the War Office. He told me that I had been posted to 6th Field Ambulance and confirmed the date already given. This was extremely useful information and very fortunate for me, as I was able to wind up my practice, inform my patients that I was joining the army and, above all, take my wife and two small children down to Hereford to my father-in-law's home.

Further luck came my way when the local hospital, The Bolingbroke Hospital on Wandsworth Common, offered me accommodation in their private block until I was called up. In due course I received my papers to report to the OC 6th Field Ambulance at the

Cambridge Hospital, Aldershot. I did this feeling very self-conscious, in a train full of servicemen, and me in my brand new uniform which was having its first outing since leaving the tailors. I was then thirty-two years old, but feeling very much like a small boy going to his first boarding school.

Aldershot seemed to arrive all too soon, and I made my way to the Cambridge Hospital and was directed to the Orderly Room. Here I met the Unit Regimental Sergeant Major, Dickie Bird, who I later learned was the senior NCO in the RAMC. He was promoted to Lieutenant Quartermaster within months. He looked at my joining papers and then said to me "Is this your first day in the Army?" I wondered at the time why he smiled at my answer, but I was soon to find out. He took me to an office marked "Commanding Officer 6th Field Ambulance" and told me to knock and then enter and give in my joining papers to the Colonel. This, after saluting with my one day old salute, I tried to do but the CO went on reading his copy of *The Times* for what seemed like hours. He then condescended to look at my documents and for an equally long time said absolutely nothing.

Although this incident happened forty-five years ago or so, I remember it vividly, for I think I have always tried to be kind and reasonable in my later life when positions have been reversed. Then came the dreaded question "What service have you, Samuel?" and when I replied "Just today, sir" there descended a longer and even more horrible silence. Eventually he spoke again, saying that I would be of no use to him at all. 6th Field Ambulance was a regular unit — that is,

I presumed, until I was posted there. I really felt that that remark needed no answer and so I remained silent.

I felt very strongly that he didn't like me at all and future events proved this hypothesis. However the feeling of dislike was mutual and remained a permanency as long as he was our Commanding Officer. Then he spoke again, telling me to go to the officers' mess and see the mess secretary, and that when I had been kitted out I was to join the unit and go on a six mile route march with them in the afternoon. Despite my rather jaded feelings I found the members of the mess very pleasant and welcoming indeed and they assured me they would see me through. I drew my kit, including a new pair of army boots. That evening my feelings towards my boots and my Colonel were as one.

I soon found out that he (the Colonel, not my boots!) had been Senior Instructor at the RAMC Depot before the War, and it was said that on the day of an important cricket match, after getting his men to mow the pitch he had ordered them to cut it even closer — with scissors. I am sure that this was an apocryphal story but I believe it. He, I am glad to say, was not typical of the other senior regular officers that I met — quite the reverse; but, as events turned out he was to remain our CO for the best part of six months. My main relief lay in the fact that I was not by any means alone in my feelings for him. He turned out to be an impossible taskmaster, unfair and unforgiving. But he taught me in those six months the rudiments of being a soldier and life eventually became bearable despite him and I shall not refer to him again. Fortunately, our second in command, Major M. Rea, was able to act as a buffer to most of the difficulties. I think he kept us from mutiny!

On the 21st September 1939 we were all confined to barracks and told that we were departing for France on the 24th September as part of the British Expeditionary Force — 2nd Division, 1st Corps. Our brigade, the sixth, consisted of the 1st Battalion the Royal Berkshire Regiment, the 2nd Battalion the Durham Light Infantry and the 1st Battalion of the Royal Welsh Fusiliers, some of the cream of the British Army at that time.

We actually crossed on the 23rd September, from Southampton to Cherbourg. It was a night crossing and uneventful. But one incident at Cherbourg stayed in my mind. One of our 3-ton lorries fell out of its rope skip and dropped about thirty or forty feet onto the quay. For a moment it stood there apparently unharmed but a second or two later it collapsed and remained like a jigsaw puzzle with all its pieces spread in hundreds of different parts along the quayside. We all thought it was very funny indeed at the time, and it did a lot to sustain our morale.

We travelled in our unit transport across northern France in an uneventful but tiring way, stopping in barns and farms en route. Unfortunately for me, having joined the unit late, I had not been vaccinated or immunised against typhoid A and B and the Colonel thought I should be done at once. Now the TAB vaccine supplied by the RAMC at that particular time gave very strong reactions, due mainly to the type of protein base that the vaccine was made up in, and succeeded in giving me a temperature varying between 101° and 103° for most of the journey.

However, I managed, and we arrived at our destination on 6th October, a village called Flines-les-Raches. This was to be our home until hostilities commenced in earnest on 10th May, 1940. The village lay between Douai and Lille and its main feature was a brewery which served as a billet for our HQ company and was roughly adapted for further use as a main dressing station for about thirty patients.

In due course we became the treatment centre for cases of scabies from 1st Corps — not a very glamorous job but a very necessary one. The treatment we used was one initiated in Sweden by Doctor Marcussen, and it was supervised by Colonel Ingram, who in peacetime was Professor of Dermatology at Leeds Infirmary. In addition we started an arduous training session in the duties of a field ambulance: practising day and night convoys, map reading, compass work and general military training. But, of course, all was based on the premise of field ambulance duty behind a more or less static front line, carrying out the classic duties known to all First War soldiers, and those training between the Wars, as a medical staging post. The first medical staging post in a brigade is the field ambulance, some fifteen to thirty minutes distance behind the Brigade and evacuating cases to a Casualty Clearing Station where major surgery could be undertaken some one to two hours or so further back. But no training or reconnaissance could be done in Belgium where our troops were to be if and when Germany invaded, because Belgium itself refused to allow Allied troops on their soil until the Germans actually attacked.

Despite this, our training was thoroughly efficient and we soon became moulded into a useful unit. Some of us went to base hospitals for specialised courses and there were many changes in personnel for one reason or another. Many officers like myself were reserve or volunteer officers and we were no longer a 'regular' unit. But despite our leadership we were a very happy mess.

We often discussed, in the early days, what the future might hold, and when and where we should be working under actual war conditions. Time went by, and oddly enough by soon after Christmas I don't remember we discussed it very much at all. However, the whole atmosphere of the mess and the unit changed in March by the welcome fact that we received a new Colonel. Training continued as usual but now with a new heart. Our new CO, Lieutenant-Colonel Jim Hyatt, turned us into a really happy and unit-proud outfit. He made our work more rational and introduced leadership with discipline and fairness and example, instead of leadership by rank and Army Orders.

Subsequent events were to show me the powers of leadership, courage and marked efficiency that our Colonel had and I owe him a deep sense of gratitude and admiration which has stayed with me long after his unfortunate death from lung disease after the war.

# II

On the 9th and 10th of May we heard air raid warnings in many neighbouring villages and the sound of distant bombing. To all of us the fact was quite clear that the so-called "phoney" period was over. I have no doubt that each of us had our own reactions, but as for mine they were of fear. For the first time since I had been in the Army I felt frightened, though I do not really know what I was frightened of. Rationalising it, I suppose I was frightened of being in a strange environment, and frightened that I would not be able to do the job I had been training for. It was a very eerie feeling, and I knew that whatever "cushiness" there had been before, it had gone, and that in vulgar parlance "we were for it".

The main dressing station had been closed some days before so we were able to put our training into effect and get ourselves ready for the journey to our new appointed destination behind 2nd Division. After an all-night move in our own transport, we found ourselves in Belgium, and we reached a large convent near Malaise, and moved in. In the morning we provided transport to help the nuns get away to what we thought at the time was safety and then we set up our first main dressing station.

Our position was just behind the River Dyle and that afternoon we received our first batch of casualties. After treating shock and re-dressing where necessary, we evacuated them via the 2nd Field Ambulance at our rear to the casualty clearing station many miles away in France. The rest of the day was uneventful, except we sent out a second company to form an advanced dressing station.

In the evening orders were received telling us to retire and just before we left we encountered the first of many problems. Some forty or fifty severely wounded men were brought in, six of them with tourniquets. Perhaps ten of the remainder were in a very sorry way. As we were not intending to move back very far we decided to take those patients with us in our own ambulances. This we did and moved back to a suburb of Brussels called Boitsfort via La Hulpe and Gronendagz. From what I saw of it, Boitsfort was very much part of the Brussels 'stockbroker belt'. Here the convoy halted on the outskirts while the Colonel reconnoitred a possible site for our main dressing station.

I seized the opportunity to enter all the ambulances and have a quick look at all our cases. They were fortunately in the main fairly comfortable, but sadly in need of medical attention, especially of course those with tourniquets.

After a wait of some quarter of an hour, the Colonel came and asked me to come with him to a nearby hotel, Hotel Haute Maison. When we entered we found this to be in a very normal state — to our absolute amazement full of guests and a dinner dance in progress. The lounge was packed and nightlife was in full swing. What shocked us most — I think all of us — was that the lounge was crowded with Belgian Officers immaculately garbed in well creased and valetted tunics, entertaining their womenfolk. It seemed incredible then that Belgian army officers were not with their units facing the Germans. In retrospect, too, one is struck by the parallel with the celebrated episode of the Duchess of Richmond's ball at Brussels at the time of Waterloo (the scene of which was only a few miles away) 125 years before.

However, the proprietor spoke fluent English and we asked him to come out to the ambulances and ask the men where and at what time they were wounded. When he received this information he realised the seriousness of the position and got his guests immediately to evacuate the hotel. In fact, the hotel was not large, but I never saw all of it, for I was quickly immersed in what became our impromptu operating theatre, and did not emerge for most of the time we were there.

We decided to use his ballroom as the room in which to place all the casualties, and to use his dining room as an operating theatre to operate on those of the urgent cases who could not wait for anything further. We also decided that freshly laundered napkins in his restaurant were almost as good as — and certainly the nearest we would get to — sterile dressings, and we found all those and used them.

Major A. Weston and I operated on all those cases that needed such treatment, aided by anaesthetics given by Captain Gittings our Dental Officer. In all, we did about twenty such operations. Contact was made with a motor ambulance convoy that afternoon and our cases were cleared some forty minutes before we were ordered to retire once more, this time undertaking a long and very tiring journey in convoy, through congested and chaotic roads, to a small place called Herinnes: we were now not far from the Franco-Belgian border.

After finding billets, we sought a welcome sleep, but it was not to be for long. After three hours we had to move again, and arrived at another village, Quatre Vents. Here, we did at least obtain a good rest before we moved again, this time to France. Our destination was Landas and again the roads were congested and harassed by German aircraft. We prepared a school there as a main dressing station but received no casualties, and in the morning moved off again to Baisieux through roads blocked by civilians and their transport. We took over a brewery there as our main dressing station. But, again, to our disappointment, we were not called on to work, and spent a miserable twenty-four hours awaiting orders either to move or to open up, listening all the time to the continuous terrible din of the battle at Tournai. We had passed through this town earlier after it had been heavily bombed. The battle for Tournai was hard, and the 6th Brigade had very heavy casualties, and the Durham Light Infantry Battalion was almost decimated.

# III

It was always during those periods of non-work that life became so difficult. Having nothing to do but just listen to battle noise and wonder about the future was very bad for morale, at least it was for mine. I found, in company with many others, that while there was actual work to be done with the wounded, one had no thoughts for anything outside. I have found, talking with my friends, that they had the same reaction when they were at home in the UK during bombing. Once they had a job to do they seemed to lose their fear.

However, during this time we did receive orders to move. But just as the first vehicle was moving off the orders were cancelled by the arrival of a breathless Staff Officer who told us to stay put for the night. In the morning we had orders to move to Templeuve-en-Pevelle and we established ourselves in a large chateau which, oddly enough, had been the German HQ in the First War. Soon after our arrival casualties turned up in fair numbers and as any scheme for evacuation was rather nebulous, once again surgery had to be tackled. By early evening we set off again, this time an exhausting journey in the La Bassée area on congested roads — a journey that took all night and the following morning.

Exhausted we arrived and were eventually billeted again on a farm at Crois Babent but moved on before midnight just a few miles to Laventie, where we took over the school for our main dressing station. During the night we did in fact receive a few casualties and it was decided to move to the shoe factory in case casualties became heavy.

It was fortunate that we did so, because at 11 o'clock at night we received some 150 cases of all sorts, and during the night we performed some 18 operations: amputations, repair of lacerated wounds and the usual gamut of injuries in war. There was a slight lull in mid-morning but then we became very busy again, not only with military cases but with civilians as well.

Several of the casualties then needed more serious surgery. In one case I resected some 18″ of small bowel, in another closed an open pneumothorax, performed suprapubic drainage, plugging of liver wounds and all the major tasks that had to be done.

Without our help there would have been no hope of any surgical aid at all. I even managed to find time to visit a local convent to see some civilian sick.

When orders came to move off we had so many cases on our hands that they made such an order impossible to comply with and we couldn't contact the Motor Ambulance Convey at all, although strenuous efforts had been made to do so. So it was decided to carry as many cases as we could back with us in our own ambulance cars, leaving one Medical Officer and 7 orderlies behind to look after the rest, planning to come back and pick them up later — which

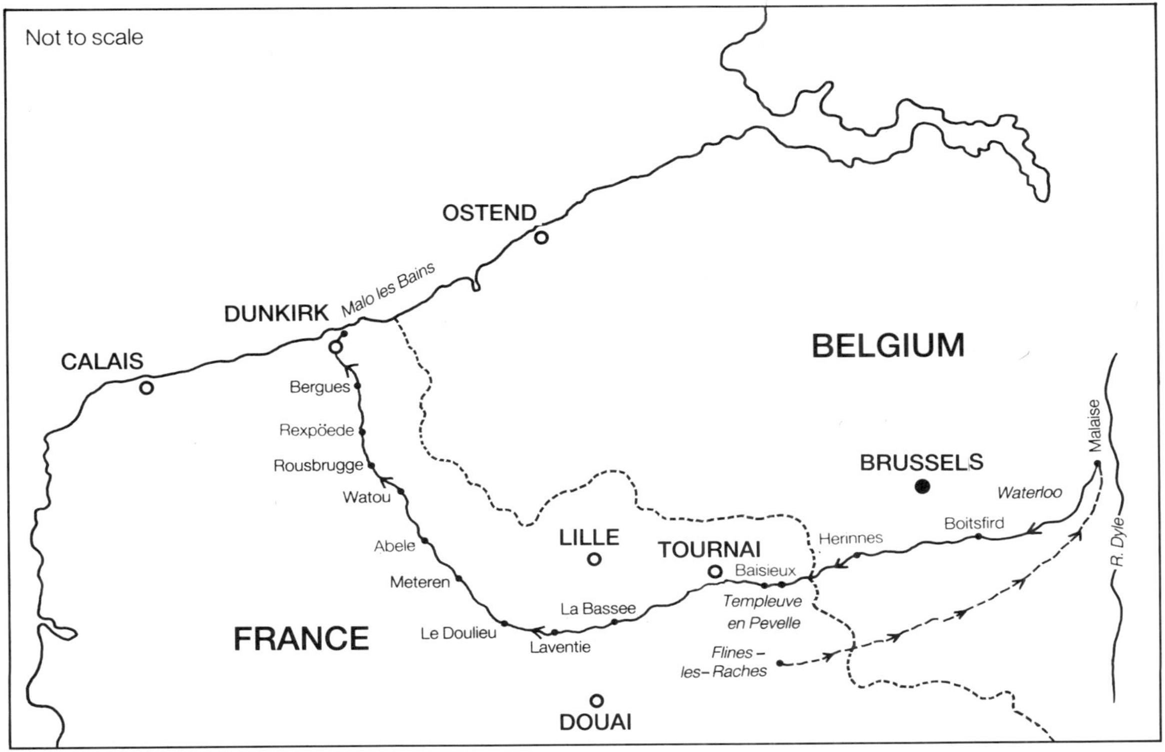
Not to scale
OSTEND
Malo les Bains
DUNKIRK
CALAIS
BELGIUM
Bergues
Rexpöede
Rousbrugge
Watou
Abele
Meteren
Le Doulieu
Laventie
La Bassee
LILLE
TOURNAI
Baisieux
Templeuve
en Pevelle
Flines –
les– Raches
Herinnes
Boitsfird
BRUSSELS
Waterloo
Malaise
R. Dyle
FRANCE
DOUAI

fortunately we were able to do, after we had moved to Le Doulieu: a very small village indeed, really consisting of two farms and their outbuildings.

There was no time to sit and admire the buildings or the lack of them because on our arrival we had to adapt it for an operating theatre immediately. Being out of touch with any other surgical unit still, on our arrival we adapted a small kitchen for use as an operating theatre and once more were able to tackle the cases which still needed surgical treatment.

Almost immediately new cases started to arrive in their dozens: French soldiers, German soldiers and French civilians, including children and of course our own wounded. These had to be placed in barns, stables and ordinary rooms, one small outhouse being reserved for those urgently injured who demanded immediate surgery.

I should say here (and perhaps I should have made it clear before), that I had myself in peacetime undergone quite considerable years of surgical training and was thus able to exercise this, because one doesn't expect when working normally with a field ambulance to have to undertake major surgery. In the normal course of events, these cases would have been sent back behind the lines to a Casualty Clearing Station where they would have received expert surgical attention. But alas we were not in contact with one. In all, in the 24 hours at Le Doulieu we received some 400–500 casualties and throughout the day and night we operated continuously in atrocious conditions. Eight amputations of leg were performed, one that of a young officer who had a compound fracture with his left leg showing the all too obvious signs of gas gangrene — a condition I had never seen before and one which, unless something was done for him, he would have died of and would almost certainly die as it was. However, we gave him his chance and amputated his leg and gave anti-gas gangrene. However he died later in the early morning and we gave him a military burial in the grounds of the farm. Apart from the poignancy of this young life dying just before us — he was only about nineteen — I remember it even better, because in the middle of burying him the German planes came over and started to fire at us and we had to abandon the funeral and go and hide in the bushes. Fortunately no one was hit and the funeral was completed.

Soon all our buildings were full up and as more and more cases arrived they had to be placed in just covered sheds, some of them more open than covered and others even had to be placed in the surrounding fields.

During these operations I got very tired and at one stage, about half way through, I had to come out and get some fresh air and then I did what I had always believed to be impossible — I fell asleep standing up. I was told that in the middle of a conversation with another member of the unit, while leaning against a barn wall, that I went sound asleep and that there was quite a few seconds without the power of legs before I fell down and woke myself up again. But I wondered then and I wondered all through the time there, with a sense of foreboding that overcame all the surgical problems, exactly how we were going to evacuate these cases because we had only given immediate treatment and they needed much more further care. We had no possible means at all of evacuating so many and we spent the remainder of the time there operating on ever increasing number of patients. Fortunately our Dental Officer and one other officer were able to give anaesthetics for me.

Some half an hour before we left Le Doulieu, a driver came into the compound with his officer who had been grossly wounded. I looked at him in the car and the whole lower half of his face had been shot away. He had no lower jaw, no lower lip or anything and looking at him one looked straight at his palate — the tongue had gone. But the horrible thing about it was he was still alive. Of course he couldn't speak — he had nothing to speak with. His eyes looked at me and moved and he moved his arms. I knew that (1) nothing could be done for him surgically and that (2) we would probably be moving quite soon, but I had to do something for him. I told the soldier to leave him and that we would do our best. He went off.

I gave this casualty a large dose of morphia and was relieved to see him become unconscious very quickly and in twenty minutes time he died, peacefully and without further trauma. Sometimes when I think back on these terrible days I see that half face and know how ghastly War can be. Some of my medical colleagues to whom I tell this story ask me how much morphia I gave him and I give you the same answer that I give to them — "I cannot remember".

# IV

At 9 o'clock the next morning we had orders to move back to Rousbrugge. This however was quite impossible because we were stuck with these hundreds of wounded and it was unthinkable that they should be left.

Then something happened which was the nearest approach to a miracle that I know. Entering the grounds of the farm was a motor ambulance convoy unit, consisting of some forty empty ambulances, lost, fed-up and depressed. In charge was a Canadian Major who had long since ceased to receive orders from anywhere and saw our unit sign outside and came in. We found him a 'home' and loaded the ambulances to capacity, in some cases cramming eighteen patients into one ambulance car and this way, I think, if my memory serves me correctly, we cleared about 420 cases and sent them on their way to Dunkirk. We had no means of finding out if they actually got to Dunkirk, but last year I contacted an orthopaedic surgeon from my own hospital, the Middlesex, Lt Col. Philip Newman, CBE, DSO, MC, F.R.C.S. — long since retired — who was famed for his exploits at twelve casualty clearing stations near Dunkirk, at Roesendael who told me in a personal communication that without doubt most of these 3–400 cases would have been processed through his casualty clearing station and evacuated on a three-hourly basis. That is, all those who were well enough to be moved. So it would seem that the miracle had worked for a very large number of our patients.

At 10 o'clock the next morning, we had orders again to move back to Rousbrugge. We took many of our fitter casualties with us, as many as we could carry — about 68 in all — leaving some 30 or 40 behind, mainly French and German wounded. Two of our orderlies volunteered to stay behind and await the arrival of the Germans, which I believe was to be only a very short time after we left. Just as we were about to leave for the journey to Rousbrugge, the Colonel and I who usually travelled in the last car at the rear of the convoy, saw a Despatch Rider coming up. He gave us the information that there were some English wounded in a village some five miles away. Colonel Hyatt decided to send Lieutenant Evans, a driver and an ambulance back to the village to collect them. The time was then about 0900 HRS in the morning on May 28th. We left then with the convoy out of sight and with us as the last vehicle of course, minus Lieutenant Evans and his ambulance. There was a slow and comparatively uneventful journey and when we nearly had reached Meteren, I saw Lieutenant Evans with his ambulance behind us, and I told the CO who stopped his car and we had a conference with Evans for some minutes, looked at his wounded and proceeded on our journey but were never able to contact the convoy again.

We travelled over the shoulder of Mont des Cats to Abele, this being an uneventful journey except for aerial bombardment of the nearby villages, especially that of Watou and when we reached there it was in flames and the road blocked by debris and tree trunks. The CO, Evans and myself partially cleared the obstructions and skirting Watou by Houtkerque, we reached the outskirts of Rousbrugge at about 14.00 HRS.

The ambulance with five lying patients and Lieutenant Evans were left in a farm while I accompanied the CO on a reconnaissance to look for our convoy. We failed in this utterly and a return was made to the farm some hours later where we remained until 17.00 HRS.

A move was then made to Oost-Capel and while waiting there we were approached by Sergeant Knight RAMC and Captain Brown of the Royal Army Service Corps of our own unit, who came to our car and told us that the convoy had been ambushed by German light tanks and armoured cars and that nearly everybody had been killed and that all those alive had been picked up by passing lorries.

Having heard this terrible news we moved on intending to contact 5th Field Ambulance. This was never possible, we never found them and proceeded to Dunkirk.

When we got back to England, there were a lot of stories going around that the Germans had never been known to fire on the Red Cross and this annoyed us as a unit very much indeed, because the attack on our field ambulance was purposeful and was obviously with the object of blocking the road so that no further traffic could come down it. We vehemently denied this story every time we heard it, and we heard it many time, but like all rumours it was told and told again and denied and denied again — I think with little effect.

Near Rexpoëde we tailed on to an enormous long traffic block until orders came to abandon vehicles and march to Dunkirk. Colonel Hyatt, Lieutenant Evans and some 15 of our men, who we had found on the way, marched with us. Shortly afterwards we noticed that our CO had disappeared. We later learnt that he had gone back with his driver to drive the ambulance patients back to Dunkirk and this he did.

In our march down the road to Dunkirk, not very far from Bergues, we saw a parachute descending with a man safely dangling at the end of it. It landed some few yards from the side of the road. We went over to him and it was a British fighter pilot whose engine had been shot in mid-air and he had had to bail out. So we told him we were making for Dunkirk and he assured us that Dunkirk was still free of the enemy, a position we were glad to have made clear for us as we really didn't have any idea whether the Germans had encircled us and got into Dunkirk. All he could think of was that about twenty minutes before he had been having a cup of tea in his mess in south Sussex. However we suggested that he should walk back with us. He found that flying boots were not really the best equipment to walk any distance in. We got into Dunkirk and were able to put him on a destroyer, as we felt that a trained pilot was a vital necessity and we should get him back to England as quickly as possible.

# V

I proceeded on foot as far as Bergues where I had to wait for some thirty minutes until the French had blown up a railway bridge, but despite taking cover I was hit in the groin by debris and after that, found walking very difficult. I proceeded on my way, accompanied now by Private Geans of the RAMC of my unit and although I now walked very laboriously, he refused to leave me and continued to help me to get along. During the course of the journey we collected at least ten stragglers and joined them on to our little party.

On entering the town of Dunkirk I made for the main quay but only French transport was seen there. The town itself was a shambles — extensively bombed and covered by a huge pall of black smoke from the burning fuel dump along the quay. In addition it was raining from a very low cloud cover, fortunately, quite unsuitable weather for aerial attack, and the visibility was equivalent to that of a very foggy day. During the time I was in the town there was no air raid, and as I was there one whole day and most of the ensuing night, it was fortuitous indeed. The only noise there was came from the not-so-distant shelling.

By this time I found it almost impossible to

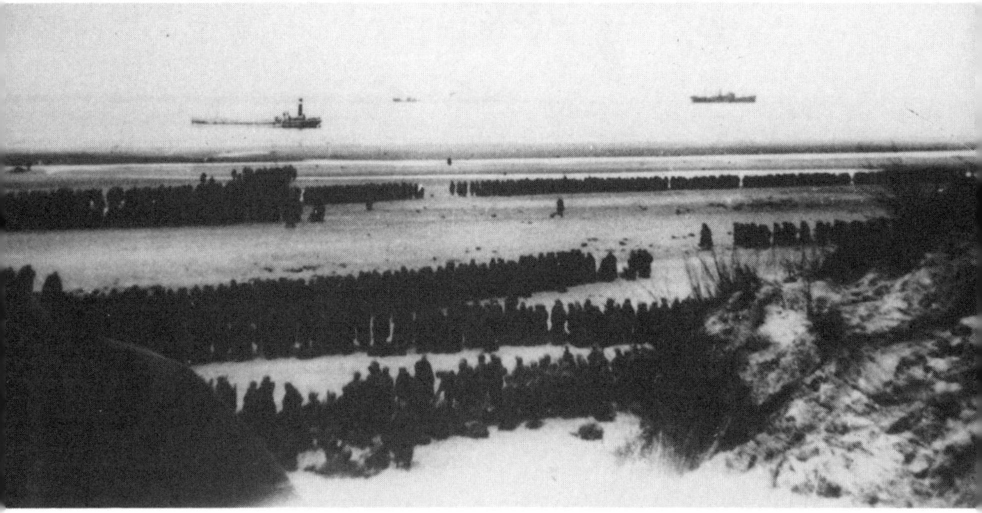

*British troops on the beach at Dunkirk.*
*(Associated Press)*

walk but Private Geans still assisted me and we made our way to some British Destroyers at the end of the quay. On reaching here I felt very ill and with hindsight I have no doubt it was due to tiredness, lack of food and drink and quite a lot of fear too and I lay down on a stretcher for some thirty minutes, after which I recovered somewhat and found Colonel Hyatt and Lieutenant Evans standing over me.

Later on that morning on 29th May we made our way to the Mole at Malo-les-Bains. We had done this on orders from a British naval officer we met on the quay. When we arrived at the Mole there was a small naval detachment in charge, and after being informed that evacuations were only taking place in the hours of darkness — owing to the previous air raids — we joined the queue.

I cannot remember much about events on the Mole itself. I think I must have slept for a large part of the time, until it was dark and the queue started to move. But I do remember Colonel Hyatt saying to me that he had received no orders to leave France and did not wish to do so. However, after a long discussion he resigned himself to the situation, but I felt very sorry for him, and can imagine what was going on in his mind.

Again my memory is hazy, but I think it was about 0400 HRS that it was my turn to embark. I can remember no feeling of relief at all, because by this time I was in a peculiar state of not thinking about anything. Events, I feel, must have overwhelmed me and I was just existing from one minute to the next. I embarked on a Dutch vessel the "Patria" and had an uneventful passage to Margate. This ship was in the command of a very young and baby-faced Sub-Lieutenant of the Royal Navy. She was a small vessel and held only about 50 of us. He asked if there was anything he could do for me and I asked if he had any food. He said no, but gave me a slug of whisky, which I think served me in better stead, for I went out like a light and when I awoke I found myself in Margate with a hangover!

At Margate, we were taken to the Dreamland, a leisure centre, and given food and drink and were then driven to Ramsgate Station where I met my Colonel and we embarked on a train for Devizes. When I say "for Devizes", I must make it clear that when we got on the train we had not the slightest idea where we were going at all.

On Ramsgate Station the Rail Transport Officer approached all troops there on the platforms and waiting rooms and thereabouts, took their names and addresses and said he would send a telegram home to next-of-kin, saying we had arrived home safely again in England. I really didn't think he would get down to such a mammoth task, but he did and my wife received his message.

From Margate we went by the train to Addison Road Station in London and got out there again for food and tea. Now Addison Road Station is, or was, the only point on the British rail system that could distribute a train to any main line throughout the whole of Britain. So they were sending trains off to their predestined places one after another.

We, of course, had no idea where we were going, but

as the journey wore on and it got darker the Colonel asked me if I had any idea of which direction we were going. I said I hadn't, but he said — looking out of the window — "I've got a feeling we're in Wiltshire". This seemed very optimistic to me. However, a little later he said "I think we're getting to my home town of Devizes" and this surprised me even more. His confidence was supreme. Within a quarter of an hour the train pulled up at a station and I looked out of the window. The notice on the platform said "Devizes" and, as if this wasn't surprising enough, there on the platform was his wife!

She had heard that there were some troops coming from Dunkirk to Devizes Station and just on the off-chance that out of all those thousands of men who were being evacuated one would be her husband, she had come to Devizes Station. Everybody of course saw them, for he was 6′ 7″ and she was 6′ 1″!

We went to the depot of the Royal Wiltshire Regiment who really laid down the red carpet for us. It was just about the middle of their weekly Mess Night and they made room for us, gave us a whopping great meal and their Commandant gave the order that the Officers should give up their beds for us and to give you some idea of my tiredness and exhaustion, I slept straight off for 16 hours.

After being re-kitted out at Devizes I was given 48 hours leave and decided I must go to Hereford and see my wife and family and intended to bring her back with me and put her up in digs at Devizes. This I managed to do but not without the most amusing experience and a forerunner of many others.

I got my taxi to Hereford alright, but in that interval of going to Hereford and seeing my family, the Government in its wisdom had decided to take down all road signposts in England to baffle any would-be invaders and my poor taximan had one hell of a job in getting back to Devizes from Hereford for lack of signposts.

But I wasn't the only Officer or Soldier thinking that I would bring my wife back to Devizes, for when we got there we could find no place for her to stay and after looking around until it got dark, the taximan said "Alright, I'll take you home" and he took us to his home and gave us a bed — which I afterwards found out was his bed, because he had only one bedroom in his flat. He gave us a splendid breakfast and refused any payment whatsoever and said "This is the sort of job I can do, being unfit for military service".

I felt considerably better after this because I'd come home rather like a dog with his tail between his legs, because I felt that (1) the Germans would be following us pretty soon and (2) we would be in disgrace in the UK. After all, the flower of the British Army had gone out in the September of 1939 to do battle with the Germans and we'd come back defeated, without arms and escaping only by the magnificence of our Navy and civilian sailors who took us out of trouble. But that was not the case: we found ourselves heroes.

I didn't look upon myself as a hero, I just felt very glad I was back alive and safe, but heroes the country made us and now Dunkirk almost ranks as one of our victories. But you can take it from me that there was no sign of victory in our 18 or 20 days or so of retreat to

Dunkirk and I still wonder what it is in the British people that makes victories out of defeat. I suppose I should have learnt a lesson from World War 1, where Mons is looked upon as a victory, although circumstances there were completely different.

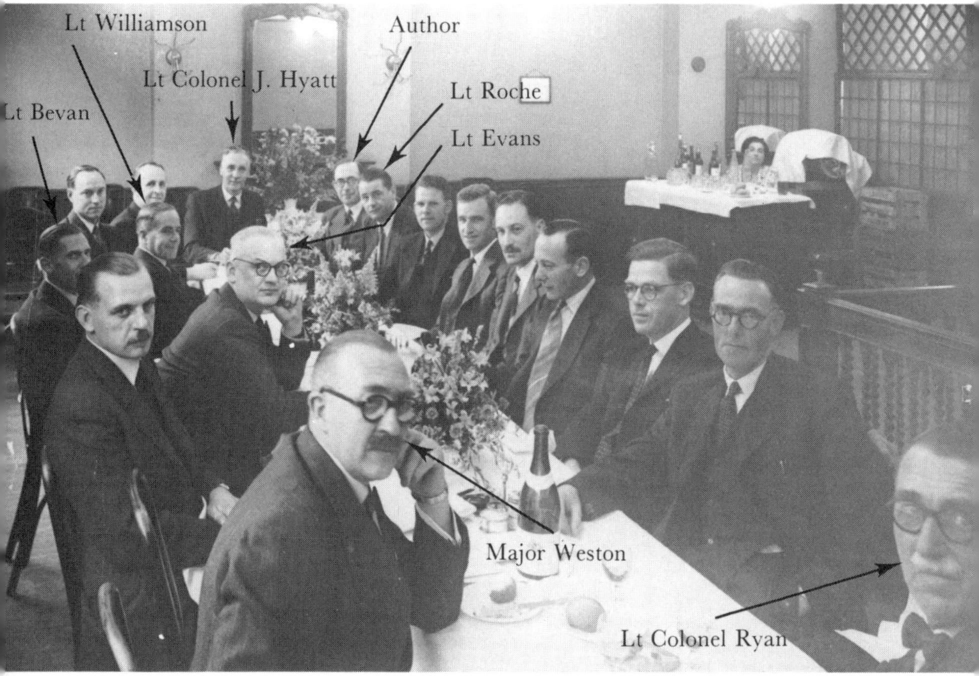


*6th Field Ambulance Officer's Reunion 1947.*

# VI

After four days at Devizes, my Colonel and I being the only members of our Unit at that depot went up, under orders, to Halifax where we met up with quite a considerable number of other ranks and two officers on the station when we got there.

The Billeting Officer put us up in the first likely-looking houses they could find. We stayed in Halifax for five days and were again treated with the utmost kindness and again, rather embarrassingly, as heroes. I got tired, like a lot of other people, of trying to tell people that we were not.

We then went to Sledmere House near Driffield in what was then the East Riding of Yorkshire and there I stayed with the unit until March 1941 and then I left them on my promotion to Major and CO of the 9th Field Hospital.

The 6th Field Ambulance in due course went out to India and Burma and acquired great fame for its conduct at the Battle of Kohima with the 2nd Division and there is great rivalry now at the re-union Dinners between those who thought that Dunkirk was their finest hour and those who were undoubtedly correct in thinking that it was Kohima.

Many people have asked me how it is that I can

remember so well so much of events during this eventful retreat. And I say that it's not odd that I should remember, it would be odd if I should ever forget. In fact, let alone forgetting, I still have occasional nightmares of certain incidents of that terrible journey to Dunkirk. Some of those incidents stick in my mind more than others.

The other thing that I remember is how I managed to do surgery with quite inadequate surgical instruments. The largest operating scalpel I had was a No. 4 size Bard-Parker and those of you who know anything about such things will realise that it is not a very big amputation knife, especially for one through the thigh. We had to borrow a carpenter's saw, and a very excellent instrument it made. We had no airways of any sort, but some thick rubber tubing with a tape through one end made an excellent substitute. Such refinements as retractors, curved forceps, needle holders — they were all absent, but nonetheless the operations were performed. Anti-Tetanic serum was given to all cases while supplies lasted and so was M & B 693, the antibiotic of those days.

Incidentally, it was only good foraging by our Quartermaster that enabled us to carry on so fully. He found, in a railway siding at Templeuve, an advance depot of medical stores with enough stores and comforts to restock three field ambulances and we took the lot.

The number of major operations numbered about 140, but we were very fortunate in the personnel of our unit for all the medical officers gave splendid anaesthetics and although the CO, Colonel Hyatt was supremely busy, he found time somehow to undertake considerable amounts of work. My two theatre orderlies, Sergeant A. Costello and Sergeant G. Edwards both worked unceasingly and without them so much work would have been impossible.

I have the greatest pleasant and pleasurable memories of my comrades, Officers and Men of the 6th Field Ambulance and I can consider myself to have been privileged to have served with them in this small portion of World War 2.

# The Second Division

FRANCE • 1939-40
ENGLAND • 1940-42
INDIA • 1942-44

THE WORLD WAR

ARAKAN • 1943
KOHIMA-ASSAM • 1944
BURMA • 1944-45

On behalf of the Commanders of the Second . . Division during the World War, I thank you

*6th British Field Ambulance*

for your service in the Division.

Our success has been largely due to the determination and devotion to duty displayed by all ranks, and we may all feel justly proud that by these successes we have maintained and enhanced the already fine record of the Second Division.

Well done. Good luck to you in your future life.

C G Nicholson.

MAJ. GEN.
COMMANDER 2ND DIVISION.

DATE *12th Sept. 1945*

# VII

# Lieutenant Colonel J. Hyatt and Sergeant E. R. Knight

The following accounts by Lieutenant Colonel J. Hyatt and Sergeant E. R. Knight confirm in general some of the events I have tried to describe.

## LIEUTENANT COLONEL J. HYATT

On the 28th May I had orders to move my Unit to an area 10 miles North West of Poperinghe and I selected Rousbrugge as a rendezvous and after seeing the convoy off, followed in my car with Lieutenant I.N. Samuel.

I had caught up and was following the last car of the convoy when Lieutenant Evans appeared with an ambulance behind my car. I stopped and ascertained that he collected wounded from a French detachment which had informed us they had some British wounded. Owing to this delay I lost touch with the convoy. On arrival at Rousbrugge I searched all the neighbourhood without finding any trace.

I later met four NCOs and men on the side of the road who informed me that the unit had been ambushed by German tanks and the vehicles burnt. They considered themselves the sole survivors.

I then proceeded until I found a Staff Officer of the 2nd Division on the road who told me that all cars were being abandoned. I later realised there would be a possibility of driving the ambulance with the wounded through. By this time I had lost touch with my other Officers, so I went down the line of transport and eventually got the ambulance down to the jetty at Dunkirk. I waited until the wounded had been loaded into a Destroyer and also found Lieutenant Duckham, my Transport Officer in another ambulance — wounded — and I saw to it that he too went with the wounded on board to be sent to the U.K.

Then Lieutenants Samuel and Evans rejoined us and we proceeded to the East Mole where we found a Naval Officer who directed us to the jetty where I embarked at about 04.30 hours on the motor barge "Senus" and disembarked at Ramsgate.

On Ramsgate Station I found Lieutenant Samuel and proceeded together with him to Devizes where, after about four days, we went to Halifax and commenced collecting the Unit with Headquarters at the Allenfield Hotel.

## SERGEANT E. R. KNIGHT

On Tuesday, 28th May the field ambulance was proceeding to a new location with ambulances full of wounded personnel followed by the remainder of the unit transport. All was going well until we passed through a place called Meteren. We ran into some enemy fire coming from a clump of trees.

I was in the back of one of the lorries with some others of my company and felt a bullet (I think it was a bullet) go through the medical pannier on which I was sitting and looking out of the back of the lorry, saw some tanks which opened fire on us setting fire to some of the lorries.

I ordered all the men to get out and we found ourselves in a ditch half-full of water and as the firing was getting worse we were not able to see what was going on through the smoke and flames coming from the burning vehicles. It looked as though the entire ambulance chain of vehicles and trucks were all alight.

We decided to crawl along the ditch until we came to another ditch which led off to the left. Myself and several others of the personnel crawled along this ditch, where we came across Staff Sergeant Fowler attending to the French interpreter who had been wounded in the back. Being unable to offer any assistance, not having any medical kit of any kind, we waited there in the hedges in the corner of the field.

We were still under fire from enemy sources, so much so that Staff Sergeant Fowler ordered me to take the other men and make our way back to separate positions and safer positions. We made our way across various fields until we came to a road and eventually came across a small convoy who gave a few of us a lift. The remainder continued to walk until they also got a lift for a couple of miles.

I then saw a vehicle with our unit mark on it and found to my surprise that it was occupied by our Colonel, Colonel Hyatt, Lieutenant Evans and Lieutenant Samuel who were absolutely stunned by the news of the disaster which had overtaken the field ambulance.

After travelling a few more miles we were stopped outside Dunkirk and made our way to the harbour on foot, as no more vehicles were being allowed in and they were being blown up. We finally arrived at Dunkirk at about 21.00 hours absolutely sopping wet through from the ditch and the rain that was pouring down outside.

I eventually rejoined my unit in Halifax where they were reforming and filling in the vacancies from the casualties.

# Index